BREAST C
COOKBOOK FOR SENIORS

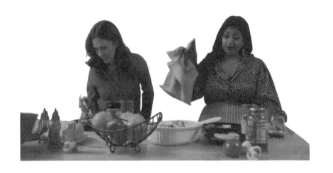

Ignite Your Recovery with Nourishing Recipes and Expert Direction

DR. SANDRA HICKS

@2023 Dr. Sandra hicks

TABLE OF CONTENT

INTRODUCTION

Once upon a time, there was a woman named Alice who was suffering from breast cancer. It had already spread and treatments weren't working. She had resigned herself to the fact that she would die soon.

Alice had a friend who recommended she try a breast cancer diet. At first, she was skeptical, but she decided to give it a try since she had nothing to lose. After just a few weeks, Alice could already feel a difference in her overall health.She was slowly but surely getting stronger. The longer she stuck with the diet, the better she felt. Eventually, her tumor had completely disappeared, and she was finally cancer-free

Alice was filled with joy. She could no longer feel the ache and discomfort that she had been suffering from for so long. She had been saved by taking a breast cancer diet.

Alice was so thankful that she decided to keep up with the diet even after she had beaten the cancer. She wanted to make sure that it never came back.Alice often told her story to anyone who would listen. She wanted to share her story and spread awareness of the effectiveness of the breast cancer diet.

Alice's story is a reminder of the power of diet and nutrition in combating illness. Although cancer is one of the most difficult diseases to beat, Alice showed that it can be done with a proper diet and a positive attitude.

What is a cancer diet?

The diet for breast cancer is very similar to the general healthy diet. This diet should include lots of fresh fruits and vegetables, whole grains, lean proteins, and healthy fats. Eating five or more servings of fruits and vegetables per day can help reduce your risk of developing cancer. It is also important to limit processed foods and sugary drinks, as well as sodium. Eating a balanced diet and drinking plenty of water will help to fight inflammation, reduce your risk of certain types of cancer, and promote overall good health. Additionally, it is important to focus on getting enough physical activity as well, which can help reduce your risk of cancer.

How can diet help during cancer treatment?

Eating a balanced and healthy diet during cancer treatment is an important part of helping your body fight the cancer and to help strengthen your body's ability to heal. Eating the right foods can help minimize side effects from chemotherapy and radiation, boost the immune system and reduce the risk of infection. Some of the most important foods to focus on are high-protein-rich foods such as eggs, nuts, legumes, fish, lean meats, and low-fat dairy products, which can help to ensure your body is getting enough fuel to help it support the healing process. Eating plenty of fruits and vegetables helps provide antioxidants which can help to boost your immune system. Foods rich in omega-3 fatty acids, such as salmon, sardines, and walnuts, can reduce inflammation. Foods that are high in fiber, such as whole grains, beans, and legumes, help to keep your digestive system regular and can help reduce nausea and other side effects. It is important to drink plenty of fluids, such as water, vegetable broth, and low-fat milk, to stay well hydrated. Staying away from processed and sugary foods can also help to support your body's healing process during cancer treatment. Lastly, consulting with a nutrition professional or

Registered Dietitian can help you design a diet to best support your specific needs throughout treatment.

Tips for following a cancer diet

1. Focus on fruits, vegetables, legumes, and whole grains. These foods provide essential vitamins, minerals, antioxidants, and fiber and may help reduce the risk of cancer.

2. Choose lean proteins such as fish, poultry, legumes, and beans over red meats.

3. Consume mostly plant-based foods, limiting processed and red meats, which are linked to an increased risk of cancer.

4. Maintain a healthy weight by limiting portion sizes and limiting added sugars and processed foods.

5. Stay hydrated by drinking at least eight glasses of water a day.

6. Avoid alcohol and limit consumption of sugary drinks such as soda.

7. Cook with healthy fats such as olive oil, nuts, and avocados.

8. Eat foods rich in antioxidants, such as fruits and vegetables, to reduce the risk of cancer.

9. Have regular check-ups with your doctor to monitor your health.

10. Get regular physical activity to support overall health and reduce the risk of cancer.

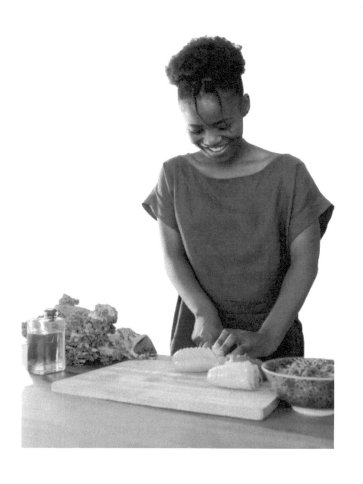

Chapter 1: Breakfast

Oatmeal with fruit and nuts

- **PREPARATION & RECIPES**

1. Gather the ingredients:

• 1 cup quick oats

• 2 tablespoons of nuts (almonds, walnuts, pecans, etc.)

• 2 tablespoons dried fruit (raisins, cranberries, etc.)

• 1–2 tablespoons honey or maple syrup

• 1–2 tablespoons butter or coconut oil

• Pinch of salt

2. Heat a medium saucepan over medium heat and melt the butter/coconut oil.

3. Once melted, add the oats, nuts and dried fruit, stirring together.

4. Pour in enough water so that the oatmeal is just submerged.

5. Add a generous pinch of salt.

6. Bring the mixture to a low boil and reduce the heat to low.

7. Let the oatmeal simmer for 3–5 minutes, stirring occasionally.

8. Add the honey/maple syrup and stir until combined.

9. Once the oatmeal has reached your desired consistency, remove from heat.

10. Serve hot with your favorite toppings!

1. Easy Banana Strawberry Oatmeal
Ingredients:
-1/2 cup rolled oats
-1 banana
-1/2 cup diced strawberries
-1/4 cup chopped nuts
-1 cup almond milk
-1/4 teaspoon salt
-1 tablespoon honey
Instructions:

1. Bring almond milk, salt, and oats to a simmer in a saucepan.

2. Once oats are softened, add banana and strawberries and reduce heat to low.

3. Cook for an additional 5 minutes.

4. Stir in nuts and honey.

2. Coconut, Apple & Cinnamon Oatmeal

Ingredients:

-1/2 cup rolled oats

-1 apple, chopped

-2 tablespoons shredded coconut

-1/4 cup chopped nuts

-1 cup almond milk

-1 teaspoon ground cinnamon

-1 teaspoon honey

-1 teaspoon vanilla extract

Instructions:

1. Bring almond milk, cinnamon, and oats to a simmer in a saucepan.

2. Once oats are softened, add apples and reduce heat to low.

3. Cook for an additional 5 minutes.

4. Stir in coconut, nuts, honey, and vanilla extract.

Yogurt with granola and berries

- **PREPARATION & RECIPES**

1. Start by measuring out your desired amount of yogurt and adding it to a bowl.

2. Top the yogurt with your desired amount of granola.

3. Next, rinse off the fresh or frozen berries of your choice and let them drain for a few minutes.

4. Add the berries to the top of the yogurt and granola.

5. Enjoy your delicious healthy snack!

1. Yogurt Parfait

Ingredients:

- 2 cups plain Greek yogurt

- 1/4 cup honey

- 1/2 cup granola

- 1/2 cup fresh berries (blueberries, strawberries, raspberries)

Instructions:

1. In a bowl, stir together 2 cups of plain Greek yogurt and 1/4 cup of honey until evenly combined.

2. Place 1/2 cup of granola in the bottom of a bowl or cup.

3. Spoon half of the yogurt mixture over the granola.

4. Top with 1/4 cup of fresh berries.

5. Repeat with remaining granola, yogurt and berries.

2. Yogurt and Granola Breakfast Bowl

Ingredients:

- 2 cups plain Greek yogurt

- 1/4 cup unsalted nuts (almonds, pecans, walnuts, etc.)
- 1/2 cup granola
- 1/2 cup fresh berries (blueberries, strawberries, raspberries)

Instructions:

1. In a bowl, stir together 2 cups of plain Greek yogurt.

2. Place 1/4 cup of unsalted nuts in the bottom of a bowl.

3. Top with 1/2 cup of granola.

4. Spoon half of the yogurt mixture over the granola and nuts.

5. Top with 1/4 cup of fresh berries.

6. Repeat with remaining granola, yogurt, nuts and berries.

Eggs with whole-wheat toast

- **PREPARATION & RECIPES**

1. Preheat a nonstick pan over medium heat.

2. Lightly spray the pan with cooking spray.

3. Crack desired amount of eggs into the preheated pan.

4. Add a pinch of salt and pepper to taste.

5. Cook the eggs, stirring occasionally, until the egg whites are solid and the yolk is still soft, about 3-5 minutes.

6. If desired, add additional ingredients, such as onion, peppers, ham, sausage, etc.

7. Toast 2 slices of whole-wheat bread until golden brown.

8. Plate the eggs with the toast and serve.

1. Huevos Rancheros:

Ingredients:

- 2 large eggs

- 2 tablespoons vegetable oil

- ¼ cup salsa

- 2 small flour tortillas

- 2 slices of whole wheat toast

- ¼ cup shredded cheese

- Salt and pepper to taste

Instructions:

1. Heat the oil in a medium-sized frying pan over medium-high heat.

2. Crack the eggs into the pan and sprinkle with salt and pepper.

3. Cook for 3-4 minutes, until the eggs are set on the bottom.

4. Carefully flip the eggs and cook for an additional 2-3 minutes, until the egg whites are set.

5. Meanwhile, warm the tortillas in the microwave for 30 seconds.

6. Toast the slices of whole wheat bread.

7. To assemble, divide the eggs between the two tortillas.

8. Top each one with salsa, cheese, and a slice of toast.

2. Healthy Egg Sandwich:

Ingredients:

-2 large eggs

-1 tablespoon butter

-2 slices of whole wheat bread

-1 tablespoon light mayonnaise

-1 tablespoon fresh chives, chopped

-Salt and pepper to taste

Instructions:

1. Heat the butter in a medium-sized frying pan over medium-high heat.

2. Crack the eggs into the pan and sprinkle with salt and pepper.

3. Cook for 3-4 minutes, until the eggs are set on the bottom.

4. Flip the eggs and cook for an additional 2-3 minutes, until the egg whites are set.

5. Meanwhile, toast the slices of whole wheat bread.

6. Spread mayonnaise on each slice of toast.

7. Divide the eggs between the two slices and top with chopped chives.

Smoothies

-

Smoothies are a great way to stay cool in the summer heat. To make a tasty smoothie, you will need a blender, frozen fruits and vegetables, liquid (e.g. almond milk, yogurt, or juice), such as honey, yogurt, or juice, and any desired add-ins (optional).

1. Gather your ingredients. Try to use at least one frozen fruit or vegetable and one liquid.

2. Cut up any larger fruits or vegetables into smaller, easy-to-blend pieces.

3. Place all ingredients in the blender. Start with the frozen fruits and vegetables. Add the liquid and any desired add-ins, and stir.

4. Blend ingredients until they are the desired consistency. If the smoothie is too thick, add

more liquid; if too thin, add more frozen ingredients.

5. Pour the smoothie into your favorite glass or mug.

1. Tropical Kale Smoothie

Ingredients:

- 1 cup kale
- 1 cup pineapple
- 1 banana
- 1/3 cup plain Greek yogurt
- 1/2 cup orange juice
- 1 Tbsp honey

Instructions:

1. Combine all ingredients into a blender and blend until smooth.

2. Enjoy!

2. Banana Berry Cup Smoothie

Ingredients:

- 1 banana

- 1/2 cup frozen mixed berries
- 2/3 cup apple juice
- 1/2 cup plain Greek yogurt

Instructions:

1. Add all ingredients to a blender and blend until smooth.

2. Enjoy!

3. Mango Coconut Smoothie

Ingredients:

- 1/2 cup mango
- 1/2 cup coconut milk
- 1/2 cup plain Greek yogurt
- 2 tsp honey

Instructions:

1. Add all ingredients to a blender and blend until smooth.

2. Enjoy!

Smoothies can be enjoyed any time of day, but they are typically most commonly enjoyed for breakfast.

Scrambled tofu with vegetable

1. Tofu Veggie Scramble

Ingredients:

-1 block extra-firm tofu, drained

-1 tablespoon sesame oil

-1 red pepper, diced

-1 onion, diced

-1 cup mushrooms, sliced

-1 garlic clove, minced

-1/4 cup low-sodium soy sauce

-3 drops liquid smoke

-1/4 teaspoon vegan Worcestershire sauce

-1/2 teaspoon smoked paprika

-1/4 teaspoon turmeric

-2 tablespoons nutritional yeast

-salt and pepper, to taste

-Veggies of your choice (peas, carrots, etc…), diced

Instructions:

1. Preheat a large nonstick skillet over medium heat.

2. Crumble the tofu into small bite-size pieces and add it to the skillet along with the sesame oil.

3. Sauté the tofu for 5-7 minutes or until it starts to brown, stirring frequently.

4. Add the red pepper, onion, mushrooms, and garlic and sauté for another 4-5 minutes.

5. Add the soy sauce, liquid smoke, Worcestershire sauce, smoked paprika, turmeric, and nutritional yeast. Stir to combine.

6. Reduce the heat to low and add the vegetables. Simmer for about 5 minutes or until the vegetables are tender.

7. Add salt and pepper, to taste. Serve warm.

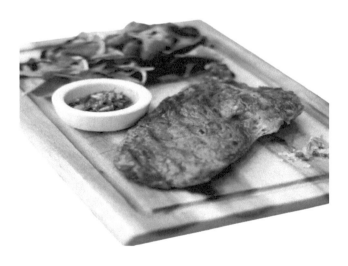

Chapter 2: Lunch

Salads with grilled chicken or fish

- **PREPARATION** & **RECIPES**

1. Grilled Southwest Chicken Salad: Start by marinating boneless, skinless chicken breasts in a mixture of lime juice, olive oil, salt, garlic, pepper, chili powder, cumin, and oregano. Then, heat a grill to medium-high heat and cook the chicken 5-7 minutes per side until cooked through. Let cool and then dice into cubes. To serve, assemble a salad that includes romaine lettuce, grilled bell peppers, black beans, corn, tomatoes, and avocado. Drizzle with a mixture of olive oil, lime juice, and honey.

2. Grilled Fish Nicoise Salad: Start by marinating the fish of your choice in a mixture of olive oil, lemon juice, garlic, salt, and pepper.

Heat a grill to medium-high heat and cook the fish for 4-6 minutes per side until cooked through. Let cool and then flake into smaller pieces. To serve, assemble a salad that includes romaine lettuce, boiled potatoes, hard boiled eggs, garlic-lemon vinaigrette, olives, and grilled vegetables.

3. Grilled Greek Chicken Salad: Start by marinating boneless, skinless chicken breasts in a mixture of oregano, olive oil, lemon juice, garlic, salt, and pepper. Then, heat a grill to medium-high heat and cook the chicken 5-7 minutes per side until cooked through. Let cool and then dice into cubes. To serve, assemble a salad that includes butter lettuce, diced cucumbers, tomatoes, feta cheese, Kalamata olives, and roasted red peppers. Drizzle with a mixture of olive oil, lemon juice, oregano, and garlic.

4. Grilled Salmon Caesar Salad: Start by marinating a salmon filet in a mixture of olive

oil, lemon juice, garlic, salt, and pepper. Heat a grill to medium-high heat and cook the salmon for 4-6 minutes per side until cooked through. Let cool and then flake into smaller pieces. To serve, assemble a salad that includes romaine lettuce, garlic-yogurt dressing, Greek yogurt, Parmesan cheese, and grilled asparagus.

5. Grilled Shrimp and Avocado Salad: Start by marinating peeled and deveined shrimp in a mixture of olive oil, lime juice, garlic, salt, and pepper. Heat a grill to medium-high heat and cook the shrimp for 2-3 minutes per side until cooked through. Let cool and then dice into cubes. To serve, assemble a salad that includes romaine lettuce, diced tomatoes, avocado, zucchini, cucumber, cilantro, and grilled pineapple. Drizzle with a mixture of olive oil, lime juice, honey, and ground cumin.

1. Grilled Chicken Salad with Bacon, Avocado & Feta

2. Grilled Fish Tacos with Cilantro Slaw

3. Grilled Chicken Caesar Salad

4. Grilled Salmon & Arugula Salad

5. Greek Salad with Grilled Shrimp

6. Grilled Chicken & Watermelon Salad

7. Grilled Tuna Nicoise Salad

8. Grilled Trout Salad with Corn & Bacon

9. Grilled Sea Bass Salad with Mango Salsa

10. Grilled Halibut & Fresh Herb Salad

Lunch time is usually around 12:00 or 1:00 pm, so I would recommend making a salad with grilled chicken or fish during this time. You could easily make a salad dressed with some greens, grilled chicken or fish, and vegetables like tomatoes, onions, or cucumbers. If you're looking for a heartier meal, you could add some grains or legumes like brown rice, quinoa, or beans, as well as nuts or seeds for some crunch and additional protein.

Soups

- **PREPARATION & RECIPES**

1. Heat oil in a large pot over medium-high heat.

2. Add diced onion, garlic, carrots, and celery and cook for about 4 minutes, stirring occasionally.

3. Add stock and bring to a simmer, then add a pinch of salt and pepper.

4. Add dried herbs such as thyme and bay leaf and stir them in.

5. Add the protein of your choice, such as diced chicken, fish, or beans (optional).

6. Simmer for 15 to 20 minutes or until the vegetables are tender.

7. Reduce heat to low and stir in any additional seasonings or ingredients like cream, noodles, or peas.

8. Cook for an additional 5 minutes or until heated through.

9. Serve in bowls and enjoy

1. Minestrone Soup
Ingredients:

- 2 tablespoons olive oil

- 1 medium onion, diced

- 3 cloves garlic, minced

- 2 carrots, peeled and diced

- 2 celery stalks, diced

- 1 can (14.5 ounces) diced tomatoes

- 1 can (15 ounces) white beans, drained and rinsed

- 2 cups vegetable stock

- 1 teaspoon dried oregano

- ½ teaspoon dried thyme

- Salt and freshly ground black pepper

- 2 cups shredded kale

- Grated Parmesan cheese, for serving

Instructions:

1. Heat olive oil in a large pot over medium heat.

2. Add the onion, garlic, carrots, and celery and cook for 5 minutes.

3. Add the tomatoes, beans, vegetable stock, oregano, thyme, salt, and pepper. Bring to a boil.

4. Reduce the heat to low and simmer, covered, for 20 minutes.

5. Add the kale and cook for another 5 minutes.

6. Taste and adjust seasonings if necessary.

7. Serve with a sprinkle of Parmesan cheese.

2. Creamy Cauliflower Soup

Ingredients:

- 2 tablespoons olive oil

- 1 onion, diced

- 2 cloves garlic, minced

- 2 heads cauliflower, cut into florets

- 4 cups vegetable broth

- 1 cup milk

- Salt and pepper, to taste

- Fresh thyme, diced, for garnish

Instructions:

1. Heat the olive oil in a large pot over medium heat.

2. Add the onion and garlic and cook for 5 minutes.

3. Add the cauliflower and vegetable broth and bring to a boil.

4. Reduce the heat to low and simmer, covered, for 20 minutes.

5. Carefully blend the soup using an immersion blender or regular blender until smooth.

6. Add the milk and season with salt and pepper.

7. Simmer for another 5 minutes.

8. Taste and adjust seasonings if necessary.

9. Ladle into bowls and garnish with fresh thyme.

3. Potato Leek Soup

Ingredients:

- 2 tablespoons olive oil

- 2 leeks, sliced and washed

- 2 large potatoes, peeled and diced

- 4 cloves garlic, minced

- 4 cups vegetable broth

- ½ cup cream

- Salt and pepper, to taste

Instructions:

1. Heat the olive oil in a large pot over medium heat.

2. Add the leeks and potatoes and cook for 5 minutes.

3. Add the garlic and cook for another minute.

4. Add the vegetable broth and bring to a boil.

5. Reduce the heat to low and simmer, covered, for 20 minutes.

6. Carefully blend the soup using an immersion blender or regular blender until smooth.

7. Add the cream and season with salt and pepper.

8. Simmer for another 5 minutes.

9. Taste and adjust seasonings if necessary.

10. Ladle into bowls and serve hot.

Lunch time is usually around 12:00 or 1:00 pm.

Sandwiches on whole-wheat bread

- **PREPARATION & RECIPES**

1) Hummus and Cucumber Sandwich: Spread a layer of hummus on two slices of whole-wheat bread. Top one slice with thinly sliced cucumber, season with salt and freshly ground black pepper, and cover with the other slice.

2) Turkey and Avocado Sandwich: Spread a generous layer of mayonnaise or Dijon mustard on two slices of whole-wheat bread. Top one slice with thickly sliced cooked turkey and avocado slices. Season with salt and freshly ground black pepper, and cover with the other slice.

3) Peanut Butter and Banana Sandwich: Spread a layer of peanut butter on two slices of whole-wheat bread. Top one slice with banana slices and a pinch of cinnamon, and cover with the other slice.

4) Apple and Cheese Sandwich: Spread a layer of apple butter on two slices of whole-wheat bread. Top one slice with thinly sliced apple and slices of mild cheese, season with salt and freshly ground black pepper, and cover with the other slice.

It depends on the person, but sandwiches on whole-wheat bread generally take anywhere from 5 minutes to 15 minutes to make.

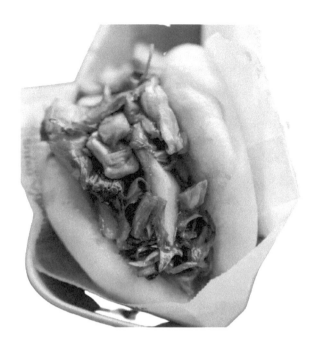

Leftovers from dinner

- **PREPARATION & RECIPES**

1. Turkey and Vegetable Fried Rice:

Ingredients:

- 2 cups leftover turkey, diced

- 2 cups cooked white or brown rice, cooled

- 2 tablespoons vegetable oil

- 1 onion, diced

- 2 carrots, diced

- 1 cup frozen peas

- 2 tablespoons soy sauce

- 2 tablespoons sesame oil

- Optional: 1 teaspoon freshly grated ginger, 2 cloves garlic, minced.

Instructions:

1. Heat the oil in a large skillet or wok over medium-high heat.

2. Add the onions and carrots and cook for 4-5 minutes, until tender.

3. Add the peas and cook for an additional 2 minutes.

4. Add the diced turkey and cooked rice and cook for an additional 4 minutes, stirring often.

5. Add the soy sauce, sesame oil, and optional ginger and garlic to the pan and mix to combine.

6. Cook for an additional 2 minutes, stirring often.

7. Serve warm.

2. Turkey Noodle Soup:

Ingredients:

- 2 tablespoons olive oil

- 2 carrots, chopped

- 2 celery stalks, chopped

- 1 onion, chopped

- 4 cups chicken or vegetable broth

- 1/2 teaspoon dried thyme

- 2 cups cooked egg noodles

- 2 cups cooked, diced turkey

- Salt, to taste

Instructions:

1. Heat the olive oil in a large pot over medium heat.

2. Add the carrots, celery, and onion and cook for 5 minutes, until tender.

3. Add the broth and thyme to the pot and bring the liquid to a boil.

4. Reduce the heat to low and simmer for 10 minutes.

5. Add the egg noodles and turkey and cook for an additional 5 minutes, stirring occasionally.

6. Season the soup with salt, to taste.

7. Serve warm.

Hummus and vegetables

- **PREPARATION & RECIPES**

Hummus:

Ingredients:

- 1 ½ cups canned cooked chickpeas
- 2-3 cloves of garlic
- 2 tablespoons tahini
- Juice of 1 lemon
- 2 tablespoons olive oil
- ¼ teaspoon salt
- ¼ cup water

Instructions:

1. Place chickpeas, garlic, tahini, lemon juice, olive oil, and salt into a food processor and blend until smooth.

2. Add the water and continue blending until desired consistency is reached.

3. Taste and adjust seasonings, if needed.

4. Serve with vegetables or crackers. Enjoy!

Vegetables:

Ingredients:

- 2 tablespoons olive oil
- 1 cup diced onions
- 1 cup diced carrots
- 1 cup diced celery
- 1 tablespoon minced garlic
- Salt and pepper to taste

Instructions:

1. Heat the olive oil in a large skillet over medium-high heat.

2. Add the diced onions, carrots, and celery. Cook for 5-7 minutes, or until vegetables are softened.

3. Add the garlic and cook for an additional 1-2 minutes.

4. Season with salt and pepper, to taste.

5. Serve with hummus and enjoy.

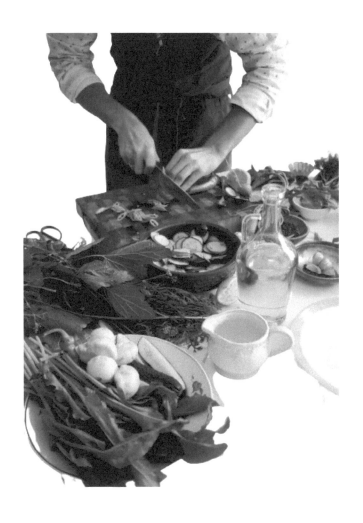

Chapter 3: Dinner

Grilled salmon with roasted vegetables

- **PREPARATION & RECIPES**

1. Preheat the grill to medium-high heat.

2. Place the salmon filets in a shallow dish.

3. In a separate bowl, toss the peppers, zucchini, and Brussels sprouts in the olive oil, and season with salt and pepper.

4. Transfer the vegetables to a greased baking sheet.

5. Grill the salmon filets for 4-5 minutes per side until cooked through.

6. Place the vegetables on the grill for 6-7 minutes, or until desired degree of doneness.

7. Drizzle the salmon and vegetables with lemon juice.

Ingredients:

- 2 salmon filets
- 1 red pepper, chopped
- 1 yellow pepper, chopped
- 1 zucchini, chopped
- 1 cup Brussels sprouts, trimmed and halved
- 2 tablespoons olive oil
- Salt and pepper, to taste
- 2 tablespoons lemon juice

Instructions:

1. Preheat the grill to medium-high heat.

2. Place the salmon filets in a shallow dish.

3. In a separate bowl, toss the peppers, zucchini, and Brussels sprouts in the olive oil, and season with salt and pepper.

4. Transfer the vegetables to a greased of baking sheet.

5. Grill the salmon filets for 4-5 minutes per side until cooked through.

6. Place the vegetables on the grill for 6-7 minutes, or until desired degree of doneness.

7. Drizzle the salmon and vegetables with lemon juice.

8. Serve immediately.

Chicken stir-fry with brown rice

- **PREPARATION & RECIPES**

1. Gather and measure all the ingredients.

2. Chop the chicken into 1-inch pieces.

3. Mince the garlic and ginger.

4. Slice the vegetables.

5. Cook the brown rice according to package instructions.

Ingredients

-4 tablespoons vegetable oil

-1 1/2 pounds boneless skinless chicken breasts, cut into 1-inch pieces

-4 cloves garlic, minced

-2 tablespoons fresh grated ginger

-2 bell peppers, any color, thinly sliced

-1 onion, diced

-3 tablespoons soy sauce

-2 tablespoons rice vinegar

-2 tablespoons brown sugar

-1 tablespoon sesame oil

-3 cups cooked brown rice

-1/4 cup cilantro, finely chopped

Instructions:

1. Heat 2 tablespoons of vegetable oil in a large skillet over medium-high heat.

2. Add the chicken and cook for 4-5 minutes, stirring occasionally, until golden and cooked through.

3. Remove the chicken from the skillet and set aside.

4. Reduce the heat to medium and add 2 tablespoons of vegetable oil.

5. Add the garlic, ginger, bell peppers, and onion and stir fry until the vegetables are tender, about 3-4 minutes.

6. Add the soy sauce, rice vinegar, brown sugar, and sesame oil and stir to combine.

7. Return the chicken to the pan and stir to combine.

8. Add the cooked brown rice and stir to combine.

9. Cook for an additional 3-4 minutes or until heated through.

10. Serve with cilantro garnish and additional soy sauce, if desired.

Lentil soup

- PREPARATION & RECIPES

Ingredients:

- 1 tablespoon olive oil
- 1 onion, chopped

- 2 cloves garlic, chopped
- 2 cups vegetable broth
- 2 cups dry lentils, rinsed
- 1 bay leaf
- 1 teaspoon dried oregano
- 1 teaspoon ground cumin
- 1 teaspoon paprika
- ¼ teaspoon cayenne pepper (optional)
- Salt and pepper, to taste
- 2 tablespoons chopped fresh parsley

Instructions:

1. Heat the olive oil in a large pot over medium-high heat. Add the onion and garlic and cook until softened, about 5 minutes.

2. Add the vegetable broth, lentils, bay leaf, oregano, cumin, paprika, and cayenne pepper. Bring to a boil.

3. Reduce the heat and simmer until the lentils are tender, about 20 minutes.

4. Discard the bay leaf and season the soup with salt and pepper.

5. Serve the soup warm, sprinkled with chopped fresh parsley.

Veggie burgers with sweet potato fries

- **PREPARATIONS & RECIPES**

1. Preheat the oven to 350 degrees F (175 degrees C).

2. Peel and cut sweet potatoes into thin sticks.

3. Place sweet potato fries on a baking sheet. Drizzle with oil and season with salt and pepper.

4. Bake in a preheated oven for 30 minutes or until golden brown.

5. In a medium bowl, mix together black beans, vegetables, and seasonings.

6. Shape mixture into small patties.

7. Heat a lightly oiled skillet over medium-high heat.

8. Cook patties for 3 to 5 minutes per side or until golden brown and heated through.

Ingredients:

- 2 sweet potatoes
- 1 tablespoon olive oil
- Salt and pepper to taste
- 1 (15 ounce) can black beans, drained and rinsed
- ½ cup diced onion
- ½ cup cooked white rice
- ½ cup shredded carrots
- ½ teaspoon garlic powder
- ½ teaspoon ground cumin
- ¼ teaspoon chili powder

Instructions:

1. Preheat the oven to 350 degrees F (175 degrees C).

2. Peel and cut sweet potatoes into thin sticks.

3. Place sweet potato fries on a baking sheet. Drizzle with olive oil and season with salt and pepper.

4. Bake in a preheated oven for 30 minutes or until golden brown.

5. In a medium bowl, mix together black beans, vegetables, and seasonings.

6. Shape mixture into small patties.

7. Heat a lightly oiled skillet over medium-high heat.

8. Cook patties for 3 to 5 minutes per side or until golden brown and heated through.

9. Serve patties with sweet potato fries. Enjoy!

Black bean tacos

- **PREPARATION & RECIPES**

1. Begin by preparing the black beans. If using dry beans, rinse them and then place them in a pot of water. Bring the water to a boil and then reduce to a simmer. Simmer for 1-2 hours or until the beans are soft and tender.

2. While the beans are cooking, you can prepare the rest of the taco toppings. Shred some cheese and cut up some tomatoes, lettuce, onions, peppers, and your favorite toppings.

3. When the beans are done cooking, drain them and place them in a bowl. Add some cumin, chili powder, garlic powder, and salt to the bowl. Stir to combine. You can also add some cilantro and lime juice for extra flavor.

4. Heat a skillet over medium heat and warm up some oil. Add the black bean mixture and cook for about 5-7 minutes, stirring frequently.

5. Warm up your tortillas in the oven or on the stove top.

6. To assemble the tacos, place a few spoonfuls of the black beans onto each of the tortillas.

Add the desired toppings and garnish with extra cilantro and lime juice if desired. Serve warm.

1. Classic Black Bean Tacos

Ingredients:

2 cups cooked black beans

1/4 cup chopped onion

1/4 cup chopped tomatoes

2 tablespoons olive oil

2 cloves garlic, minced

1 teaspoon ground cumin

1 teaspoon chili powder

1/4 teaspoon salt

8 soft taco shells

1/2 cup crumbled queso fresco

Salsa, for serving

Instructions:

1. In a medium skillet, heat the olive oil over medium heat. Add the onion, garlic, cumin,

chili powder, and salt. Cook and stir until the onion is soft, about 5 minutes.

2. Add the cooked black beans and tomatoes to the skillet. Cook and stir until the black beans are warmed through, about 5 minutes.

3. Place a spoonful of the black bean mixture into each taco shell. Top with optional crumbled queso fresco and salsa. Serve.

2. Mexican Black Bean Tacos

Ingredients:

2 tablespoons vegetable oil

1 onion, chopped

3 cloves garlic, minced

2 tablespoons chili powder

1 teaspoon cumin

1/2 teaspoon dried oregano

1/4 teaspoon cayenne pepper

2 cups cooked black beans

4-6 soft taco shells

1 (11-ounce) package pre-shredded Mexican cheese blend

1 avocado, mashed

1/2 cup diced tomatoes

1/4 cup chopped fresh cilantro

Fresh lime wedges, for serving

Sour cream, for serving

Instructions:

1. In a medium skillet over medium heat, heat the vegetable oil. Add the onion and garlic and cook until the onion is softened, about 4 minutes.

2. Add the chili powder, cumin, oregano, and cayenne to the skillet and cook, stirring often, for 1 minute.

3. Add the cooked black beans to the skillet and cook, stirring often, until heated through, about 5 minutes.

4. Place a spoonful of the black bean mixture into each taco shell. Top with Mexican cheese

blend, mashed avocado, tomatoes, cilantro, and optional lime wedges and sour cream.

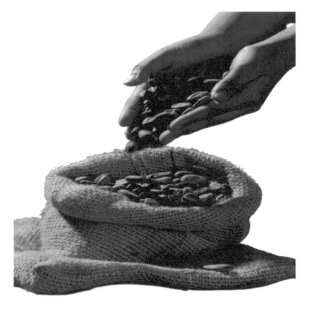

Chapter 4: Snacks

Fruits and vegetables

- **PREPARATION & RECIPES**

1. Gather your ingredients. Make sure to have a variety of fruit and vegetables available.

2. Wash all fruits and vegetables with cold water.

3. Cut fruits and vegetables into small, bite-sized pieces.

4. Place all pieces in the refrigerator to chill until ready to use.

5. Preheat the oven to 375 degrees.

Recipe 1: Baked Zucchini Chips

Ingredients:

• 2 medium zucchini

• 1 tablespoon olive oil

• ¼ teaspoon each of garlic powder, onion powder, salt, and pepper

Instructions:

1. Slice the zucchini into thin chips, about 1/8" thick.

2. Place the zucchini slices onto a baking sheet lined with parchment paper.

3. Brush the zucchini slices with olive oil.

4. Sprinkle the zucchini chips with garlic powder, onion powder, salt, and pepper.

5. Bake for 20 minutes, flipping halfway through.

2. Roasted Carrot Chips

Ingredients

• 2 large carrots

• 2 teaspoons olive oil

• ¼ teaspoon each of salt, pepper, and garlic powder

Instructions

1. Preheat the oven to 375 degrees.

2. Slice the carrots into thin coins, about 1/8" thick.

3. Place the carrot slices on a baking sheet lined with parchment paper.

4. Brush the carrots with olive oil.

5. Sprinkle carrots with salt, pepper, and garlic powder.

6. Bake for 20 minutes, flipping halfway through.

Nuts and seeds

- PREPARATION & RECIPES

1. Savory Sunflower Seed Mix

Ingredients:

- 2 cups raw sunflower seeds
- 2 tablespoons olive oil
- 1 teaspoon garlic powder
- 1 teaspoon onion powder
- 1/4 teaspoon sea salt
- 1/4 teaspoon smoked paprika

Instructions:

1. Preheat the oven to 350 degrees Fahrenheit and line a baking sheet with parchment paper.

2. In a small bowl, combine the olive oil, garlic powder, onion powder, sea salt and smoked paprika.

3. Add the sunflower seeds to the mix and stir until all the seeds are evenly coated.

4. Spread the seeds onto the lined baking sheet in a single layer.

5. Bake in the preheated oven for 20-25 minutes, stirring at the 10 minute mark.

6. Remove from the oven and let cool. Enjoy!

2. Coconut Cashew Protein Bites

Ingredients:

- 1/2 cup cashew butter
- 1/4 cup honey
- 1/4 cup ground flaxseed
- 1/3 cup shredded coconut
- 1/4 cup hemp seeds
- 1/2 teaspoon ground cinnamon
- 1/4 teaspoon sea salt

Instructions:

1. In a medium bowl, combine the cashew butter, honey, flaxseed, coconut, hemp seeds, cinnamon and sea salt.

2. Mix until all ingredients are well combined.

3. Take about 1 tablespoon of the mixture and roll into a ball.

4. Place the ball on a parchment-lined baking sheet.

5. Continue the process until all the mixture has been used.

6. Place the baking sheet into the freezer for 1 hour.

7. Store in an air-tight container in the refrigerator.

Yogurt

- PREPARATION & RECIPES

1. Gather the ingredients. You will need plain, unflavored yogurt and any desired flavorings such as fresh or frozen fruit, honey, sugar, vanilla, cocoa powder, spices, or jam.

2. Place the yogurt in a bowl and mix in the desired flavorings.

3. Add the mixture to a food processor and process for 1-2 minutes, or until the desired consistency is reached.

4. Place the mixture in air-tight containers or molds.

5. Refrigerate the mixture for at least 2 hours before serving.

Recipes

1. **Blueberry Honey Yogurt**: Blend together plain yogurt, 1 cup of fresh or frozen blueberries, 1 tablespoon of honey, and 1 teaspoon of vanilla extract in a food processor. Refrigerate overnight before serving.

2. **Chocolate Banana Yoghurt**: Blend together plain yogurt, 1 banana, 3 tablespoons of cocoa powder, 1 tablespoon of sugar, and 1/2 teaspoon of cinnamon in a food processor. Refrigerate overnight before serving.

3. Mango Peach Yoghurt: Blend together plain .
yogurt, 1 mango, 1 peach, 1 tablespoon of
honey, and 1 teaspoon of sugar in a food
processor. Refrigerate overnight before serving.

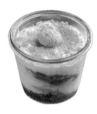

Hard-boiled eggs

- **PREPARATION & RECIPES**

1. Gather the necessary ingredients: eggs, a pot
for boiling, a bowl of ice water, and a slotted
spoon.

2. Fill the pot with enough cold tap water to
cover the eggs completely.

3. Place the pot on the stovetop and set the burner to high.

4. When the water boils, use the slotted spoon to delicately lower the eggs into the pot.

5. Boil the eggs for 10 minutes.

6. Once the eggs have finished boiling, remove the pot from the stovetop and strain the eggs from the water using the slotted spoon.

7. Place the eggs in a bowl of ice water for 10 minutes to allow for easy peeling.

1. Hard Boiled Eggs with Garlic Mayo

Ingredients:

- 4 hard boiled eggs, peeled and halved lengthwise
- 1/4 cup mayonnaise
- 2 cloves of garlic, minced
- Salt and pepper to taste

Instructions:

1. In a small bowl, mix together the mayonnaise, minced garlic, salt, and pepper.

2. Spread the garlic mayonnaise over the halved hard boiled eggs.

3. Serve cold.

2. BLT Egg Salad

Ingredients:

- 4 hard boiled eggs, peeled and chopped
- 1/2 cup diced bacon
- 1/4 cup mayonnaise
- 1/4 cup diced tomato
- 1/4 cup diced red onion
- Salt and pepper to taste

Instructions:

1. In a medium bowl, combine the chopped eggs, bacon, mayonnaise, tomato, and red onion.

2. Mix until everything is combined.

3. Season with salt and pepper and mix to combine.

4. Serve on top of toasted bread or in a wrap.

Trail mix

- **PREPARATION & RECIPES**

Trail Mix Recipe #1:

Ingredients:

- 1/2 cup dry-roasted peanuts

- 1/2 cup walnuts pieces

- 1/4 cup sunflower seeds

- 1/4 cup pumpkin seeds

- 1/2 cup raisins

- 1/2 cup dark chocolate chips

Instructions:

1. In a large bowl, combine the dry-roasted peanuts, walnut pieces, sunflower seeds, pumpkin seeds, and raisins.

2. Toss the mixture to combine.

3. Add the dark chocolate chips and mix until everything is evenly distributed.

4. Place the trail mix in zipper plastic bags or a storage container for easy transport.

Trail Mix Recipe #2:

Ingredients:

- 1/2 cup almonds
- 1/2 cup cashews
- 1/4 cup dried cranberries
- 1/4 cup dried cherries
- 1/2 cup banana chips
- 1/2 cup dark chocolate chips

Instructions:

1. In a large bowl, combine the almonds, cashews, dried cranberries, and dried cherries.

2. Toss the mixture to combine.

3. Add the banana chips and dark chocolate chips and mix until everything is evenly distributed.

4. Place the trail mix in zipper plastic bags or a storage container for easy transport.

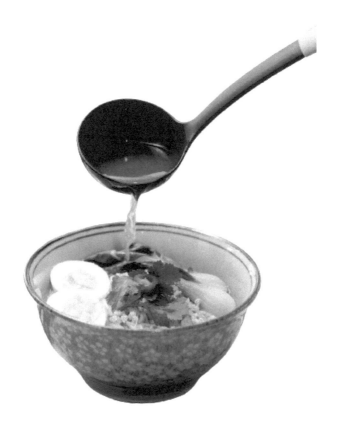

Chapter 5: Desserts

Fruit salad with yogurt

- **PREPARATION & RECIPES**

Fruit Salad with Yogurt

Ingredients:

- 2 cups mixed fresh fruit (such as diced apples, berries, grapes, and other diced fruits of your choice)
- 1/4 cup plain yogurt
- 2 teaspoons honey
- 1 tablespoon freshly-squeezed orange juice
- 1/4 teaspoon ground cinnamon

Instructions:

1. In a large bowl, combine the diced fruit.

2. In a separate bowl, whisk together the yogurt, honey, orange juice, and cinnamon.

3. Pour the yogurt mixture over the fruit and stir to combine.

4. Refrigerate for at least 10 minutes before serving.

Frozen yogurt

- **PREPARATION & RECIPES**

Frozen Yogurt

Ingredients:

-4 cups plain nonfat yogurt

-1/4 cup sugar

-2 teaspoons vanilla extract

-1/2 cup of your favorite fruit, diced (optional)

Instructions:

1. In a large bowl, stir together the yogurt, sugar, and vanilla extract until blended.
2. Optional: Add the diced fruit to the mixture and stir.
3. Pour the mixture into an ice cream maker and follow the manufacturer's instructions for churning.
4. When the yogurt reaches a soft-serve consistency, transfer to a container with a lid and freeze for at least two hours before serving.

Frozen Yogurt Popsicles
Ingredients:

-2 cups plain nonfat yogurt

-1/4 cup sugar

-2 teaspoons vanilla extract

-1/4 cup diced fruit (optional)

-Popsicle molds

Instructions:

1. In a medium bowl, stir together the yogurt, sugar, and vanilla extract until blended.

2. Optional: Add the diced fruit to the mixture and stir.

3. Carefully spoon the mixture into Popsicle molds and insert sticks.

4. Freeze for at least three hours before serving.

Popsicles

- **PREPARATION & RECIPES**

1. Watermelon Strawberry Popsicles
Ingredients:
- 2 cups watermelon, cubed
- 2 cups strawberries, hulled
- 1/4 cup fresh lime juice
- 2 tablespoons sugar

Instructions:
1. Place the watermelon, strawberries and lime juice in a blender. Blend until smooth.

2. Pour the mixture into popsicle molds and sprinkle with the sugar.

3. Place the molds in the freezer and freeze for at least 4 hours or until solid.

4. Enjoy your Watermelon Strawberry Popsicles!

2. Chocolate Banana Popsicles

Ingredients:
- 2 bananas, peeled and sliced
- 1 cup plain yogurt
- 2 tablespoons cocoa powder
- 2 tablespoons honey

Instructions:

1. Place the bananas, yogurt, cocoa powder and honey in a blender. Blend until smooth.

2. Pour the mixture into popsicle molds.

3. Place the molds in the freezer and freeze for at least 4 hours or until solid.

4. Enjoy your Chocolate Banana Popsicles!

Chocolate avocado mousse

- **PREPARATION & RECIPES**

Chocolate Alvarado Mousse

Ingredients:

- 2 cups semi-sweet chocolate chips
-2 tablespoons of butter
-1/4 teaspoon of sea salt
-3/4 cup of heavy cream
-1 tablespoon of sugar
-1 teaspoon of vanilla extract
-3 egg yolks
-1/4 cup of Alvarado St. Bakery Sprouted Bread crumbs

Instructions:

1. In a medium saucepan, melt the chocolate chips, butter, and sea salt together over low heat; stirring constantly until the mixture is fully melted and completely blended together.
2. Remove the pan from the heat and transfer the chocolate mixture to a large bowl to cool.

3. Whip the heavy cream until stiff peaks form; set aside.

4. In a separate bowl, whip together the egg yolks, sugar, and vanilla extract until light and fluffy.

5. Fold the whipped egg yolks into the cooled chocolate mixture. then gently fold in the whipped cream.

6. Pour the mousse into 6 individual serving dishes. Top each dish with Alvarado St. Bakery sprouted bread crumbs.

7. Refrigerate the mousses for 3 hours before serving.

Pumpkin bread

- **PREPARATION & RECIPES**

Pumpkin Bread
Ingredients:

- 2 cups all-purpose flour
- 2 teaspoon ground cinnamon
- 2 teaspoon baking powder
- 1 teaspoon baking soda
- 1 teaspoon salt
- 2 cups granulated sugar
- 4 large eggs
- 1 cup (2 sticks) butter, melted
- 2 cups canned pumpkin
- 1/2 cup chopped walnuts (optional)

Instructions:

1. Preheat the oven to 350°F. Grease a loaf pan with baking spray.

2. In a medium bowl, combine the flour, cinnamon, baking powder, baking soda and salt.

3. In a large bowl, beat the sugar, eggs and butter until light and fluffy.

4. Add the canned pumpkin and mix until combined.

5. Gradually add the flour mixture into the wet ingredients and mix until just combined.

6. Gently fold in the walnuts (if desired).

7. Pour the batter into the prepared loaf pan and bake for 1 hour or until a toothpick inserted into the center of the loaf comes out clean.

8. Let cool in the pan for 10 minutes, then turn out onto a cooling rack to cool completely.

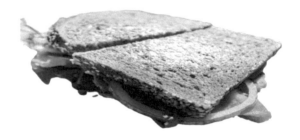

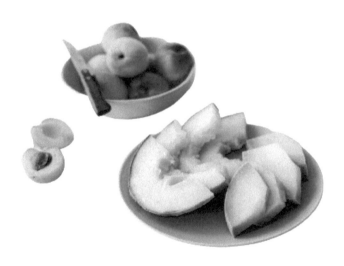

APPENDIX

In addition to the breast cancer diets recipes provided in this cookbook, this appendix provides further information about nutrition for seniors with breast cancer.

1. Supplements: Many people over the age of 65 are recommended to supplement their diet with vitamins and minerals, especially vitamin D, calcium, and Omega-3 fatty acids. Your doctor can help you determine which supplements are right for you.

2. Food Groups: Eating a well-rounded diet is important for people of all ages, but especially seniors with breast cancer. Focus on a diet that contains foods from all major food groups, including fruits, vegetables, lean proteins, whole grains, low fat dairy, and healthy fats.

Aim for 5-9 servings of fruits and vegetables every day.

3. Hydration: Staying hydrated is critical for everyone, but especially for seniors. Drink 8 glasses of water or other non-alcoholic fluids each day, and more if you are feeling thirsty or active.

4. Portion Sizes: As we age, our appetite tends to decrease and our body does not need as many calories. Keep your portions small and try to stick to a regular eating schedule.

5. Calorie Needs: Your specific calorie needs depend on your age, size, activity level, and health. Talk to your doctor or registered dietitian to find out how many calories you should be eating every day.

We hope this cookbook and its associated appendix have provided you with useful information about nutrition and lifestyle for seniors with breast cancer. With these tips, you can make informed choices that help you nourish your body and stay healthy.

RESOURCES FOR CANCER PATIENTS AND THEIR FAMILIES

- Cook Without a Book: Meatless Meals by Pam Anderson
- Quick and Healthy Recipes and Ideas by Brenda Ponichtera
- The Cancer-Fighting Kitchen: Nourishing, Big-Flavor Recipes for Cancer Treatment and Recovery by Rebecca Katz with Mat Edelson
- Fresh and Healthy Cooking for Cancer Survivors: Easy and Delicious Recipes and Tips for Those With Cancer and Their Caregivers by Sarah Schlesinger and Richard Schlesinger
- The Cancer-Fighting Cookbook: Over 200 Recipes and Nutrition Strategies for Preventing and Surviving Cancer by Rebecca Katz

Support Groups

• The Wellness Community
• CancerCare
• American Cancer Society
• Cancer.Net Support Groups
• National Coalition for Cancer Survivorship
Financial and Emotional Resources

• Cancer Financial Assistance Coalition
• National Association of Hospital and Health Care (NAHCH)
• Cancer Patient Navigators
• CaringBridge
• National Coalition for Cancer Survivorship

Online Resources
• Cancer.Net
• The American Cancer Society
• National Cancer Institute
• Cancer Research UK
• Cancer Care
• Livestrong

SPECIAL RECIPES FOR DIET

1. Maple Pecan Oatmeal Pancakes:
Ingredients:

-2 cups all-purpose flour

-3/4 cup quick cooking oats

-2 teaspoon baking powder

-1 teaspoon baking soda

-1/2 teaspoon ground cinnamon

-1/4 teaspoon salt

-2 cups buttermilk

-1/4 cup pure maple syrup

-1/4 cup brown sugar

-2 eggs, lightly beaten

-1/4 cup butter, melted

-1/2 cup chopped pecans

Directions:

1. In a large bowl, whisk together the flour, oats, baking powder, baking soda, cinnamon and salt.

2. In a separate medium bowl, whisk together the buttermilk, maple syrup, brown sugar, eggs and melted butter until combined.

3. Pour the wet ingredients into the dry ingredients and whisk until just combined. Do not overmix.

4. Stir in the chopped pecans.

5. Heat a large skillet or griddle over medium heat. Grease with butter or cooking spray.

6. Drop the pancake batter by 1/4 cupfuls onto the preheated skillet.

7. Cook until bubbles form on the top and the edges are slightly golden, about 2 minutes. Flip and cook until the other side is golden brown, about 2 minutes more.

8. Repeat with the remaining batter.

9. Serve warm with butter and syrup.

2. Sweet Potato Casserole

Ingredients:

- 4 large sweet potatoes

- 3 tablespoons butter

- 2 tablespoons brown sugar

- 2 tablespoons honey

- 1/2 teaspoon cinnamon

- 1/4 teaspoon nutmeg

- 1/4 teaspoon salt

- 1/2 cup slivered almonds

Instructions:

1. Preheat the oven to 350°F.

2. Peel and cut the sweet potatoes into bite-sized cubes. Place in a large pot and cover with water and bring to a boil. Cook for 10 minutes until soft.

3. Drain the potatoes and mash with butter, brown sugar, honey, cinnamon, nutmeg and salt.

4. Spread mixture into a greased baking dish. Sprinkle with almonds.

5. Bake for 20 minutes or until golden brown.

3. Cranberry Brie Tart

Ingredients:

- 2 tablespoons butter

- 1 sheet ready-made puff pastry, thawed

- 1 wheel brie

- 1/2 cup cranberry sauce

Instructions:

1. Preheat the oven to 400°F.

2. Cut the puff pastry into a 14-inch circle and place on a baking sheet lined with parchment paper.

3. Spread butter on the pastry.

4. Slice the brie and place the slices on top of the pastry.

5. Top with the cranberry sauce.

6. Bake for 25 minutes until golden brown.

7. Let cool before serving.

4. Cranberry & Brie Stuffed Turkey Breast

Ingredients:

- 2 lb turkey breast, deboned

- 4 oz Brie Cheese, cut into small cubes

- ½ cup dried cranberries

- 2 tbsp olive oil

- 2 tbsp fresh rosemary, chopped

- Salt and pepper, to taste

Method:

1. Preheat the oven to 375°F.

2. Pat the turkey breast dry with a paper towel and season with salt and pepper.

3. Place turkey breast in a baking dish.

4. In a small bowl, mix together Brie cheese, dried cranberries, olive oil, and chopped rosemary.

5. Stuff the mixture into the turkey breast and spread it evenly.

6. Cover the baking dish with aluminum foil and bake for 50 minutes, or until the internal temperature reads 165°F.

7. Let the turkey rest for 10 minutes before slicing and serving.

5. Sweet Potato & Squash Latkes

Ingredients:

- 1 large sweet potato, grated
- ½ yellow squash, grated
- 1 onion, grated
- 2 eggs, beaten
- 2 tbsp all-purpose flour
- 2 tbsp chopped fresh chives
- 2 tbsp olive oil
- Salt and pepper, to taste

Method:

1. In a large bowl, mix together grated sweet potato, squash, onion, eggs, flour, chives, and salt and pepper.

2. In a large skillet, heat the olive oil over medium heat.

3. Once the oil is heated, spoon in the batter and press it into small patties.

4. Cook for about 2 minutes, or until golden brown and crispy. Flip and cook the other side for an additional 2 minutes.

5. Transfer to a paper towel-lined plate and serve.

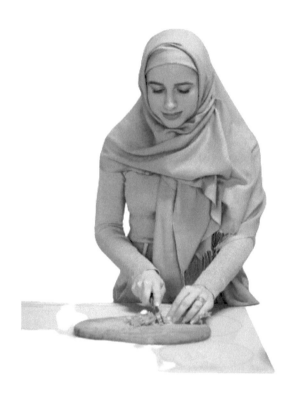

Made in United States
Troutdale, OR
07/26/2023

11575930R00056